Statement on the Scope and Standards of Oncology Nursing Practice

Editors
Jeannine M. Brant, RN, MS, AOCN®
Rita S. Wickham, PhD, RN, AOCN®, CHPN

Authors
Deborah A. Boyle, RN, MSN, AOCN®, FAAN
Susan D. Bruce, RN, BSN, OCN®
Ryan R. Iwamoto, ARNP, MN, AOCN®
Barbara L. Summers, PhD, RN

Field Reviewers
Cheryl A. Bean, DSN, APRN, BC, AOCN®, ANP
Carol S. Blecher, RN, MS, AOCN®, APN, C*
Carol Curtiss, RN, MSN
Elaine C. Glass, RN, MS, APRN, BC-PCM
Linda A. Jacobs, PhD, RN, AOCN®
Lisa Schulmeister, RN, MN, CS, OCN®

Oncology Nursing Society
Pittsburgh, PA

ONS Publishing Division
Publisher: Leonard Mafrica, MBA, CAE
Director, Commercial Publishing/Technical Editor: Barbara Sigler, RN, MNEd
Production Manager: Lisa M. George, BA
Staff Editor: Lori Wilson, BA
Graphic Designer: Dany Sjoen

Statement on the Scope and Standards of Oncology Nursing Practice

ISBN 1-890504-49-1

The Oncology Nursing Society acknowledges the American Nurses Association for their contribution to this edition and previous editions of the *Statement on the Scope and Standards of Oncology Nursing Practice*.

Printed in the United States of America

Oncology Nursing Society
Integrity • Innovation • Stewardship • Advocacy • Excellence • Inclusiveness

Contributors

Editors

Jeannine M. Brant, RN, MS, AOCN®
Oncology Clinical Nurse Specialist and Pain Consultant
St. Vincent Healthcare
Billings, Montana

Rita S. Wickham, PhD, RN, AOCN®, CHPN
Clinical Nurse Specialist, Section of Palliative Care
Associate Professor of Nursing
Rush University Medical Center
Chicago, Illinois

Authors

Deborah A. Boyle, RN, MSN, AOCN®, FAAN
Practice Outcomes Nurse Specialist
Banner Good Samaritan Medical Center
Phoenix, Arizona

Susan D. Bruce, RN, BSN, OCN®
Clinical Nurse IV
Department of Radiation Oncology
Duke University Medical Center
Durham, North Carolina

Ryan R. Iwamoto, ARNP, MN, AOCN®
Oncology Clinical Coordinator
Genentech BioOncology
Seattle, Washington

Barbara L. Summers, PhD, RN
Vice President and Chief Nursing Officer
Head, Division of Nursing
University of Texas M.D. Anderson Cancer Center
Houston, Texas

Field Reviewers

Cheryl A. Bean, DSN, APRN, BC, AOCN®, ANP
Associate Professor
Indiana University School of Nursing
Indianapolis, Indiana

Carol S. Blecher, RN, MS, AOCN®, APN, C*
Advanced Practice Nurse, Clinical Manager
Hematology and Oncology Associates of New Jersey, LLC
Union, New Jersey

Carol Curtiss, RN, MSN
Clinical Nurse Specialist Consultant
Curtiss Consulting
Greenfield, Massachusetts

Elaine C. Glass, RN, MS, APRN, BC-PCM
Clinical Nurse Specialist
Palliative Care at Grant Medical Center
Columbus, Ohio

Linda A. Jacobs, PhD, RN, AOCN®
Clinical Assistant Professor
Coordinator, Living Well After Cancer Program
Abramson Cancer Center of the University of Pennsylvania
Philadelphia, Pennsylvania

Lisa Schulmeister, RN, MN, CS, OCN®
Oncology Nurse Consultant
New Orleans, LA

The Oncology Nursing Society would like to thank the following individuals for their work on the previous edition of this publication (credentials reflect those listed in the 1996 publication).

Editor
Jeannine M. Brant, MS, RN, OCN®, AOCN®

Authors
Ryan R. Iwamoto, MN, ARNP
Kimberly A. Rumsey, MSN, OCN®
Barbara L. Young Summers, PhD, RN, CS

ANA Liaison
JoAnn Disch, PhD, RN, FAAN

Reviewers
Cheryl A. Bean, DSN, RN, CS, AOCN®
Carol P. Curtiss, MSN, RN, OCN®
Elaine C. Glass, MS, RN, OCN®
Nancy A. Hayes, MS, RN, OCN®
Judith A. Kostka, MS, RN, MBA
Esther Muscari Lin, MSN, RN, AOCN®
Noella D. McCray, MN, RN, OCN®
Patricia A. Morris, MSN, RN, OCN®, CNA
Kathleen M. Shuey, MS, RN, AOCN®, CS
Cherie L. Tofthagen, RN, OCN®

Special Thanks To:
The Coalition of Psychiatric Nursing Organizations

Table of Contents

Preface

The development of nursing standards has been a strong emphasis of the American Nurses Association (ANA) since the late 1960s, and the ANA published the first nursing standards of practice in 1973. These introductory standards were generic in nature and focused on the nursing process. The standards were the impetus toward quality nursing care. Shortly thereafter, many nursing organizations developed standards of practice specific to the various specialty practices that exist within the nursing profession. In 1979, the Oncology Nursing Society (ONS), in collaboration with ANA, published *Outcome Standards for Cancer Nursing Practice*. A second collaborative effort in 1987 led to the development of the *Standards of Oncology Nursing Practice*, and this document was revised in 1996 to form the *Statement on the Scope and Standards of Oncology Nursing Practice* (ANA & ONS, 1996).

This publication reflects the dynamic evolutionary changes that are present in oncology nursing practice. The focus of this document, consistent with the historical versions, describes the role of the professional oncology nurse. The 2004 *Statement on the Scope and Standards of Oncology Nursing Practice* includes the following:

- The historical foundation and contemporary changes that exist within the oncology nursing profession
- The "Scope of Oncology Nursing Practice" that recognizes oncology nursing as a nursing specialty
- The "Standards of Care" that reflects professional nursing activities described through the nursing process; the 11 high-incidence problem areas in the 1996 document have been expanded to 14, with the inclusion of complementary and alternative therapies, palliative and end-of-life care, and survivorship consistent with current practice
- The "Standards of Professional Performance" that emulates professional nursing activities that lie outside of the nursing process; the focus areas have been expanded from the 1996 document to include leadership and to further define practice evaluation and education of the professional nurse.

This document reflects the goals of ONS to promote the highest quality of care in persons at risk for cancer, experiencing cancer, and/or surviving cancer.

Introduction

Foundation for Oncology Nursing

Reflecting on health care in the 20th century, there has been tremendous progress in cancer care and the development of oncology nursing as a subspecialty. In this new era, there is opportunity to look ahead at the challenges and opportunities of oncology nursing in the 21st century.

Since publication of the previous edition of these standards (1996), a series of phenomena has occurred that has significantly challenged health care, cancer care, and oncology nursing. These phenomena are the result of several key shifts in the demographics of the U.S. population, including the growing number of elderly individuals, increasing racial and ethnic diversity, and the rising number of uninsured individuals (National Center for Health Statistics, 2002). In addition, aging individuals commonly experience one or more chronic health problems. These factors, when coupled with increased consumer requests for advanced healthcare technology and services, have resulted in a significant increase in demand and expenditures for health care (Institute of Medicine [IOM], 2001a).

Contemporary with the development of these challenges, professional oncology nursing practice has progressed in an environment that examines every nurse in his or her daily practice. What remain constant are the driving forces that necessitated the development of oncology specialty nursing, which focuses on the human responses of individuals and families experiencing, at risk for developing, or surviving cancer. These forces include

- The needs of individuals with cancer, at risk for developing cancer, or surviving cancer or those dying of cancer or its treatment
- National and international recognition of cancer as a major chronic health problem
- Advances in science and technology allowing expanded treatment options

- Changes in the perceptions of cancer within lay and professional publics
- A culture that denies death as a natural part of life and views death as a failure of the healthcare system
- Changes in the scope of practice and focus of the nursing profession (ANA & ONS, 1996).

Prior to the 1950s, the major cancer treatment modality was surgery, and the nurse's role was limited to inpatient care of the hospitalized surgical patient. As chemotherapy and radiation therapy became treatment modalities in the 1950s and 1960s, nurses continued to identify opportunities to contribute to the care of persons with cancer.

It was not until the 1970s that major advances occurred in the areas of cancer treatment and oncology nursing. The National Cancer Act of 1971 provided impetus for a comprehensive program focused on reducing the incidence, morbidity, and mortality of cancer. During the same time that cancer survival rates improved, nursing experienced a shift that combined expanded roles with acknowledgment of the importance of professionalism in nursing. The result was nursing involvement in educational conferences and programs that focused on oncology nursing as a specialty area in cancer care.

ONS had its inception as a result of one of these conferences and in 1975 was incorporated with the goal of promoting the highest professional standards for oncology nurses. ONS has developed an organizational structure and has created resources to support this goal. These resources include the *Statement on the Scope and Standards of Oncology Nursing Practice*.

Contemporary Issues and Trends

Advances in oncology nursing practice parallel and contribute to advances in cancer prevention, diagnosis, treatment, and survivorship. As oncology nursing has furthered the development of a body of professional knowledge grounded in research and practice, nurses are evermore playing central roles in each aspect along the cancer care continuum. Overall cancer incidence rates remained stable in the United States from 1995 to 1999, whereas cancer death rates steadily declined in all age groups from 1993 to 1999, possibly because cancer is more likely to be diagnosed and treated at earlier stages (Edwards et al., 2002; Ries et al., 2003). Progress in cancer survival has been associated with the development of more effective treatment approaches and more aggressive use of improved supportive care interventions, as well as cancer prevention and control activities. Oncology nurses have been at the forefront of these advances, particularly in the areas of prevention and detection. As the number of cancer survivors increases, oncology nurses also are providing leadership in supporting the unique needs of this population.

Three recently identified contemporary issues have significant implications for oncology nurses. First, IOM published a series of reports detailing deficiencies in healthcare quality and patient safety (IOM, 2001a, 2001b, 2003; Kohn, Corrigan, & Donaldson, 2000). Second, the American Hospital Association (2002) and other professional organizations cite research that warns about an impending long-term shortage of healthcare workers and the impact of this shortage on healthcare delivery services. Third is the IOM position on improving care at the end of life.

According to IOM, " The American health care delivery system is in need of fundamental change. Many patients, doctors, n urses, and health care leaders are concerned that the care delivered is not, essentially, the care we should receive" (IOM, 2001a, p. 1). Recommendations in the IOM report *Crossing the Quality Chasm* explicitly address the roles and responsibilities of healthcare professionals in raising the quality of care (IOM, 2003). These include a recommendation that professional groups ". . . pursue six major aims; specifically, healthcare should be safe, effective, patient-centered, timely, efficient, and equitable" (IOM, 2001b, p. 7). Other recommendations resonate with oncology nursing standards of practice, such as that healthcare providers should redesign the processes of care to be based on continuous healing relationships consistent with patient needs and values, apply evidence-based decision making to standardize practices, and actively collaborate and communicate to coordinate care. In

2003, IOM elucidated necessary competencies to meet patient needs in the 21st century, including delivering patient-centered care, functioning as interdisciplinary team members, and using evidence-based practices to improve the quality of care. The current *Statement on the Scope and Standards of Oncology Nursing Practice* contains both standards of care and standards of professional performance that provide oncology nurses with a framework to respond to the IOM challenges.

Both immediate and long-term healthcare workforce shortages, including nurses, have been described. The current shortage of healthcare workers has led to increases in the time to recruit into vacancies. The long-term shortages may be the more serious source of concern for oncology nurses because the demands for cancer care services will increase in coming years, while the existing workforce will age and the rate of growth of the labor force declines (American Hospital Association, 2002; Health Resources and Services Administration, 2002). These forces may jeopardize oncology nurses' ability to deliver quality cancer care. The *Statement on the Scope and Standards of Oncology Nursing Practice* (ANA & ONS, 1996) provides nurses and institutions with benchmarks for care and professional performance, which may be used to support practitioners' efforts to meet these challenges.

Changes in the Roles of Oncology Nurses

Oncology nursing practice has continued to evolve to meet the needs of persons throughout the cancer experience, from prevention and screening through rehabilitation and supportive care, end-of-life, and survivorship, as needed. Gains in new knowledge about cancer and cancer care are paralleled by evolving oncology nursing roles in health promotion, health protection, cancer prevention, cancer treatment, and the management of the physical, psychosocial, and spiritual effects of cancer and cancer treatment. The standards contained in this document reflect the responsiveness of oncology nursing in developing roles in cancer prevention and early detection, genetic counseling, treatment of disease, side effect management, cancer survivorship, end-of-life care, and rehabilitation. The standards also reflect an emphasis placed on collaboration, collegiality, ethics, diversity awareness and cultural competence, quality of care, and resource utilization, consistent with the changing roles of the oncology nurse, diminishing of resources, and demands of the healthcare delivery system.

Changes in Care Delivery Settings

The *Statement on the Scope and Standards of Oncology Nursing Practice* reflects the spectrum of care delivery settings in which oncology nurses practice. As cancer therapies have become more aggressive, patients receiving these therapies have become more acutely ill, often requiring critical care. This has motivated oncology nurses to e xpand their knowledge and work in specialized oncology critical care areas. Furthermore, our society is increasingly embracing the concept of end-of-life care, and oncology nurses are expanding their knowledge of palliative and end-of-life care.

Another healthcare change in the United States is the shift to ambulatory treatment. Patients who once received cancer chemotherapy in the hospital are now receiving complex treatment and care as outpatients. Furthermore, patients may no longer travel long distances to comprehensive cancer centers, but instead receive chemotherapy and symptom management in rural clinics staffed by generalist nurses. Radiation therapy options are expanding, and radiation treatment centers are found in rural areas to meet patient needs and increase the number of patients treated. Such changes in care delivery settings create opportunities for education and expansion in oncology nursing practice while emphasizing the need for consistent standards in oncology nursing practice.

Diversity Awareness and Cultural Competence

Finally, the revised standards are written to reflect an ongoing emphasis on the importance of culturally competent oncology nursing practice. The demographics of the U.S. population are shifting dramatically, with remarkable increases in the number of ethnic minority, elderly, and economically disadvantaged persons with cancer. Nursing care that is provided to patients and families along the cancer continuum must be sensitive to needs that arise from unique cultural, spiritual, ethnic, and racial factors present in each care situation. Oncology nursing practice is enriched through this diversity and always reflects respect for each unique cultural background of the patient and family. This respect also extends to appreciating the rich tapestry that is woven from the diversity found within professional colleagues.

Scope of Oncology Nursing Practice

The recognition of cancer as a major health problem has led to the development of oncology nursing as a specialty. The practice of oncology nursing encompasses the roles of direct caregiver, educator, consultant, administrator, and researcher; it extends to all care delivery settings in which patients experiencing or at risk for developing cancer receive health care, education, and counseling. The primary goals of oncology nursing practice are to promote cancer prevention and early detection practices and to facilitate optimal individual and family functioning throughout the disease trajectory.

The oncology nurse achieves these primary goals by diagnosing and treating human responses of patients and families with cancer diagnoses or who are at risk for developing cancer. These human responses include (but are not limited to) physical symptoms, functional limitations, psychosocial disruptions, and knowledge needs associated with the diagnosis and treatment of cancer and/or factors known to increase cancer risk. Treatment of these responses involves the delivery of cancer therapies and restorative physical care to manage disease and treatment-related symptoms; health promotion and disease prevention counseling; health maintenance education; psychosocial support to build or sustain coping capacity; and education to encourage active participation in decision making and self-care. Oncology nursing care is patient-centered and may encompass individuals, families, groups, and communities.

Oncology nursing practice occurs along a continuum of care and across care delivery settings. The nature of nursing care spans the spectrum from preventive and acute care through rehabilitative and palliative supportive care as necessary. Each of these subspecialties of oncology nursing care may be provided in a variety of settings: inpatient, ambulatory, hospice, home care, and long-term care.

Oncology Nursing Practice

In addition to the basic educational preparation required to function as a registered professional nurse, oncology nursing practice at the generalist level requires a cancer-specific knowledge base and demonstrated clinical expertise in cancer care beyond that acquired in a basic nursing program.

The oncology nurse functions as a coordinator of patient care, collaborating with other cancer care providers and health team members to provide high-quality care. The oncology nurse acts as a patient guide and advocate by assisting patients and families to seek information, ensuring informed consent regarding treatment decisions and promoting the maximal level of patient-desired independence.

The oncology nurse is accountable for delivering care within the framework of the nursing process. Data gathering is focused in 14 high-incidence problem areas: health promotion, education, coping, comfort, nutrition, complementary and alternative therapies, protective mechanisms, mobility, gastrointestinal and urinary function, sexuality, cardiopulmonary function, oncologic emergencies, palliative and end-of-life care, and survivorship. The oncology nurse uses assessment data to formulate nursing diagnoses and to prioritize problems according to patient need. The oncology nurse collaborates with the patient to set mutual goals to develop a plan of care directed toward achieving these identified goals. The effectiveness of the care plan in meeting goals is evaluated through measurable patient outcomes. The "Standards of Care" further delineates the 14 high-incidence problem areas and is included in the following section of this document.

The oncology nurse actively participates in professional role development activities, including quality assessment and improvement, practice evaluation, professional education, collegiality, interdisciplinary collaboration, and the review and clinical application of research findings. In addition, the oncology nurse develops ethically sound practice and confronts ethical challenges, uses resources wisely, and assumes a leadership role in health care's evolving future through application of the "Standards of Professional Performance" included in the last section of this document.

Advanced Oncology Nursing Practice

Advanced oncology nursing practice requires substantial theoretical knowledge in oncology nursing and proficient use of this knowledge in providing expert care to individuals diagnosed with cancer and their families, as well as the at-risk community-at-large. Advanced practice may include the roles of direct caregiver, coordinator, consultant, educator, researcher, and administrator (ONS, 2003). Consistent with the ANA's social policy statement and the National Council of State Boards of Nursing statement on advanced practice nursing, advanced nursing practice in oncology requires a minimum of a master's degree (ANA, 1995a, 1995b, 1996; National Council of State Boards of Nursing, 2002).

Oncology nurses practicing at the advanced level "integrate both medical and nursing paradigms and perspectives that in turn benefit the care of patients with cancer and their families" (ONS, 2003, p. 1). They must be able to assess, conceptualize, diagnose, and analyze complex clinical and nonclinical problems related to the actual or potential diagnosis of cancer. In addition, advanced practice implies the ability to consider a wide rage of theories and research relevant to understanding cancer-related problems, as well as to select and justify applying the most meaningful theory or research in problem solving.

Advanced nursing practice in oncology is actualized through various roles. The direct caregiver role requires mastery of the nursing process and the ability to provide, guide, and evaluate nursing practice delivered to individuals diagnosed with cancer, their families, and the community. The coordinator role includes expert use of the change process with the interdisciplinary cancer care team to determine and achieve realistic healthcare goals for a particular patient or for an entire community and guiding the patient through the healthcare system.

As a consultant, the advanced practice oncology nurse provides expertise about oncology to colleagues, allied health personnel, and all healthcare consumers. In the educator role, an advanced practice nurse assesses the learning needs of the patient or community and designs, implements, and evaluates educational activities. At the advanced level, the researcher role requires at least beginning research skills, such as identifying current researchable problems in cancer nursing, collaborating in research, and evaluating and implementing research findings applicable to cancer care or cancer nursing. The administrative role involves using leadership skills and the managerial process to support an environment conducive to optimal professional nursing practice.

Advanced oncology nursing practice is best defined as expert competency and leadership in the provision of care to individuals with an actual or potential diagnosis of cancer. The *Statement on the Scope and Standards of Advanced Practice Nursing in Oncology* is published in a separate document (ONS, 2003).

Standards of Oncology Nursing Practice

These standards describe the responsibilities for which oncology nurses are accountable. The framework provided by the standards describes a competent level of professional performance and professional nursing practice shared by nurses engaged in the delivery of cancer care. The "Standards of Oncology Nursing Practice" consists of two sections: "Standards of Care," which focuses on the 14 high-incidence problem areas of cancer care, and "Standards of Professional Performance." The content of each of these sections is as follows.

Standards of Care

The "Standards of Care" pertains to professional nursing activities demonstrated through the nursing process, which includes assessment, diagnosis, outcome identification, planning, implementation, and evaluation. The nursing process is the foundation of clinical decision making and encompasses all significant action taken by nurses in providing oncology care to all patients.

Standards of Professional Performance

The "Standards of Professional Performance" describes competent, professional nursing behaviors and includes activities related to quality of care, practice evaluation, education, collegiality, ethics, collaboration, research, resource utilization, and leadership. All oncology nurses are expected to engage in professional role activities based on their education, position, and practice setting. Therefore, the measurement criteria identify a broad range of activities that demonstrate compliance with the professional performance standard.

Although professional performance standards describe expected roles for all professional nurses, many other responsibilities comprise the hallmarks of professional nursing. The nurse should be self-directed and purposeful in seeking the necessary knowledge and skills to enhance professionalism. Other desirable methods of enhancing professionalism include membership in a professional nursing organization, specialty certification, and further academic education.

Conclusion

The "Standards of Oncology Nursing Practice" delineates the professional responsibilities of oncology nurses engaged in clinical cancer practice regardless of care setting. These standards serve as a basis for

- Job descriptions, performance appraisals, and peer review
- Educational offerings
- Determination of healthcare reimbursement
- Healthcare agency policies, procedures, and protocols
- Consumer evaluation of quality of nursing care
- Encouraging research to validate practice
- Development and evaluation of nursing service delivery systems and organizational structures
- Quality assessment and quality improvement systems
- Health policy development
- Regulatory agency review.

Ongoing transformations in the healthcare environment mandate that oncology nurses ensure competent clinical practice and promote ongoing professional development. This *Statement on the Scope and Standards of Oncology Nursing Practice* serves to assist oncology nurses in meeting this mandate by defining, elucidating, and reviewing the practice of oncology nursing.

References

American Hospital Association. (2002). *In our hands. How hospital leaders can build a thriving workforce.* Chicago: Author.

American Nurses Association. (1995a). *Advanced practice nursing: A new age on health care.* Washington, DC: Author.

American Nurses Association. (1995b). *Nursing's social policy statement.* Washington, DC: Author.

American Nurses Association. (1996). *Scope and standards of advanced practice registered nursing.* Washington, DC: Author.

American Nurses Association & Oncology Nursing Society. (1996). *Statement on the scope and standards of oncology nursing practice.* Washington, DC: American Nurses Publishing.

Edwards, B.K., Howe, H.L., Ries, L.A.G., Thun, M.J., Rosenberg, H.M., Yancik, R., et al. (2002). Annual report to the nation on the status of cancer, 1993–1999, featuring implications of age and aging on the U.S. cancer burden. *Cancer, 94,* 2766–2792.

Health Resources and Services Administration. (2002). *Projected supply, demand and shortages of registered nurses: 2000–2020.* Retrieved July 25, 2003, from http://bhpr.hrsa.gov/healthworkforce/rnproject/default.htm

Institute of Medicine. (2001a). *Envisioning the national health care quality report.* Washington, DC: National Academy Press.

Institute of Medicine. (2001b). *Health professions education: A bridge to quality.* Washington, DC: National Academy Press.

Institute of Medicine. (2003). *Crossing the quality chasm: A new health system for the 21st century.* Washington, DC: National Academy Press.

Kohn, L.T., Corrigan, J.M., & Donaldson, M.S. (Eds.). (2000). *To err is human. Building a safer health system.* Washington, DC: Institute of Medicine, National Academy Press.

National Center for Health Statistics. (2002). *Health, United States, 2002. With chartbook on trends in the health of Americans.* Hyattsville, MD: Author.

National Council of State Boards of Nursing. (2002). *Regulation of advanced practice nursing: 2002 National Council of State Boards of Nursing position paper.* Retrieved April 13, 2004, from http://www.ncsbn.org/pdfs/APRN_Position_Paper2002.pdf

Oncology Nursing Society. (2003). *Statement on the scope and standards of advanced practice nursing in oncology.* Pittsburgh, PA: Author.

Ries, L.A.G., Eisner, M.P., Kosary, C.L., Hankey, B.F., Miller, B.A., Clegg, L., et al. (Eds.). (2003). *SEER cancer statistics review, 1975–2000.* Retrieved July 25, 2003, from http://seer.cancer.gov/csr/1975_2000

Standards of Care

Standard I. Assessment

The oncology nurse systematically and continually collects data regarding the health status of the patient.

Rationale

Effective communication skills; physical, psychosocial, spiritual/religious, and cultural assessment skills; and review of pertinent health records help the oncology nurse determine the strengths, resources, and needs of the patient. This process allows the oncology nurse to plan appropriate interventions with the patient.

Measurement Criteria

The oncology nurse
1. Collects pertinent objective and subjective data in a timely, ongoing, systematic, and culturally competent manner.
2. Collects data from multiple sources, including the patient, the family, the interdisciplinary cancer care team members, and the community using appropriate assessment techniques.
3. Uses theoretical and evidence-based concepts in nursing to assess individual patient populations.
4. Collects data in the following 14 high-incidence problem areas that may include but are not limited to
   a. Health promotion
      1) Environmental risk factors
      2) Personal risk factors, including genetic factors
      3) Health promotion (prevention) practices
      4) Early detection practices
      5) Cultural and social factors

    b. Patient/family education
        1) Patient/family developmental and educational levels
        2) Patient/family current knowledge of diagnosis, treatment, resources, and potential problems and side effects
        3) Patient/family participation in care (e.g., financial/reimbursement issues, availability of caregivers, cultural factors, current health-related practices, palliative care)

    c. Coping
        1) Past and present coping mechanisms
        2) Past and present social support for the patient and family
        3) Effective coping strategies as identified by the patient
        4) Present concerns (e.g., physiological, psychosocial, religious or spiritual issues, role changes, changes in employment)
        5) Present and potential support systems within family and community (e.g., local community support groups, faith community)
        6) Patient/family knowledge of advance directives
        7) Ability to use available resources
        8) Effectiveness of social support and other resources
        9) Alternative coping strategies during all phases of the care continuum

    d. Comfort
        1) Location, intensity, and exacerbating and relieving characteristics of discomfort/pain and other deleterious symptoms (e.g., fatigue, nausea, dyspnea, pruritus)
        2) Methods of pain and symptom management, including cultural and folk remedies and complementary therapies
        3) Impact of pain and other distressing symptoms on daily living
        4) Effects of disease, treatment, and therapy on lifestyle
        5) Evaluation of interventions to alleviate pain and other symptoms

    e. Nutrition
        1) Baseline nutritional status
        2) Past and present nutritional patterns and beliefs

3) Effects of disease and treatment on nutrition
4) Estimated time period that patient will be at risk for nutritional impairment
5) Function of gastrointestinal tract
6) Need for alternative route for alimentation
f. Complementary and alternative medicine
   1) Patient/family beliefs about and use of complementary and alternative therapies, including cultural and folk remedies
   2) Current and past use of complementary and alternative therapies
   3) Side effects associated with use of complementary and alternative therapies
   4) Potential interactions between allopathic and complementary and alternative therapies and contraindications to complementary and alternative measures
g. Protective mechanisms
   1) Immune function
   2) Hematopoietic function
   3) Integumentary function
   4) Neurologic function, including sensory and motor function, level of consciousness, and thought processes
h. Mobility
   1) Past and present level of mobility
   2) Risk for decreased mobility
   3) Impact of fatigue on mobility
   4) Complications related to decreased mobility
i. Gastrointestinal and urinary function
   1) Past and present patterns of bowel and bladder elimination
   2) Risk for impaired bowel function (e.g., constipation, diarrhea, ileus, bowel obstruction)
   3) Effects of disease, treatment, and side effects of therapy on gastrointestinal and urinary function
   4) Nausea and vomiting
j. Sexuality
   1) Past and present sexual patterns and expression

  2) Effects of disease and treatment (e.g., alopecia, mastectomy, amputation, ostomy) on body image

  3) Effects of disease and treatment on sexual function (e.g., infertility, impotence, early menopause, decreased vaginal secretions with dryness, decreased libido)

  4) Psychological response of patient and partner to disease and treatment

 k. Cardiopulmonary function

  1) Preexisting concomitant cardiac or pulmonary disease(s)

  2) History of exposure to respiratory contaminants

  3) Alterations in tissue perfusion

  4) Alterations in cardiac output

  5) Alterations in respiratory status or gas exchange related to disease and treatment

 l. Oncologic emergencies (e.g., sepsis, spinal cord compression, hypercalcemia, tumor lysis syndrome, superior vena cava syndrome)

  1) Patients at high risk for oncologic emergencies

  2) Early signs and symptoms of impending oncologic emergencies

  3) Pertinent laboratory, radiographic, and physical findings related to oncologic emergencies

  4) Patient/family understanding about signs and symptoms to report

  5) Patient/family understanding about management of oncologic emergencies

 m. Palliative and end-of-life care

  1) Patient/family understanding about the philosophy and practice of palliative care along the entire disease trajectory

  2) Evidence of control of physical symptoms (e.g., pain, dyspnea, fatigue, nausea, anorexia) associated with serious chronic illness

  3) Benefits and side effects associated with palliative therapies

  4) Current advance directives

5) Evidence of control of physical symptoms (e.g., pain, dyspnea, nausea, delirium) associated with end-of-life care

6) Evidence of psychosocial support (e.g., support system of friends and family) versus psychosocial suffering (e.g., depression, difficulty with role changes, relationship strain) at the end of life

7) Evidence of spiritual resources (e.g., chaplain, minister, spiritual leader) or spiritual suffering (e.g., fear of the unknown, hopelessness, unresolved issues about God or a higher power)

8) Resources needed (e.g., caregiver resources, admission to hospice) to provide optimal end-of-life care

n. Survivorship

1) Patient/family understanding of the potential late effects of cancer treatment (e.g., secondary malignancies, organ toxicities, altered fertility) prior to the initiation of therapy

2) Patient/family understanding of the potential persistent changes (e.g., fatigue, taste changes, cognitive changes) associated with cancer treatment

3) Patient/family understanding of the need for adherence to long-term follow-up

5. Uses appropriate evidence-based assessment techniques and instruments in collecting data.

6. Communicates assessment data in a timely manner with appropriate members of the interdisciplinary cancer care team.

7. Documents the initial and ongoing assessment data clearly and concisely in a retrievable form, which allows for continuity of care.

Standard II. Diagnosis

The oncology nurse analyzes assessment data to determine nursing diagnoses.

Rationale

Nursing diagnoses provide the framework for identifying expected outcomes, as well as for planning, implementing, and evaluating the health concerns of patients. (The Appendix contains examples of nursing diagnoses commonly used in oncology practice.)

Measurement Criteria

The oncology nurse

1. Determines nursing diagnoses and potential problem statements from assessment data.
2. Formulates nursing diagnoses that conform to an accepted classifications system (e.g., North American Nursing Diagnosis Association, 2001).
3. Develops individualized nursing diagnoses that are physically, psychosocially, spiritually, and culturally appropriate to the patient.
4. Ensures nursing diagnoses reflect the patient's actual or potential health problems, including actual or potential alterations in the 14 high-incidence problem areas.
5. Validates nursing diagnoses with the patient, family, and interdisciplinary cancer care team when possible.
6. Prioritizes nursing diagnoses according to actual or potential threat to patient.
7. Records nursing diagnoses to facilitate their use in the plan of care and to identify expected patient outcomes.
8. Uses evidence-based research to formulate the plan of care.

Standard III. Outcome Identification

The oncology nurse identifies expected outcomes individualized to the patient.

Rationale

The identification of expected health outcomes, developed in collaboration with the patient, enables the nurse to formulate a plan of care that will meet the patient's goals. These outcomes include health promotion and maintenance, restoration, rehabilitation, or a peaceful and comfortable death.

Measurement Criteria

The oncology nurse
1. Derives expected outcomes from the nursing diagnoses.
2. Ensures that expected outcomes are physically, psychosocially, spiritually, and culturally appropriate to the patient.
3. Develops expected outcomes collaboratively with the patient, family and interdisciplinary cancer care team when possible.
4. Ensures that expected outcomes are realistic in relation to the patient's present and potential capabilities.
5. Designs expected outcomes to maximize the patient's functional abilities.
6. Formulates expected outcomes in congruence with other planned therapies.
7. Ensures that expected outcomes provide direction for continuity of care.
8. Assigns a realistic time period for expected outcomes for achievement or re-evaluation.
9. Documents expected outcomes as measurable goals based on current evidence-based research.
10. Identifies expected outcomes with careful consideration of risks, benefits, costs, current evidence-based practice, and clinical knowledge.
11. Develops expected outcomes for each of the 14 high-incidence problem areas within a level consistent with the patient's physical, psychosocial, and spiritual capacities, cultural background, and value system. The expected outcomes include but are not limited to
    a. Health promotion
       The patient and/or family
       1) Recognizes factors that place an individual at risk for and may lead to cancer, such as tobacco use, improper nutri-

tion, use of immunosuppressive agents, exposure to carcinogens, exposure to sun, aging, and genetic predisposition (e.g., familial breast cancer, skin cancer, familial polyposis, retinoblastoma, neuroblastoma, Wilms' tumor).

2) Describes the warning signs of cancer.

3) Identifies and describes specific health-promoting activities (e.g., smoking cessation), appropriate diet, and early detection methods (e.g., clinical breast examination, breast self-examination, mammography, cervical screening, testicular self-examination, skin assessment, oral self-examination, colorectal and prostate screening).

4) Identifies a plan for seeking healthcare assistance whenever any alteration in health status occurs.

5) Identifies where services can be obtained.

b. Patient/family education

The patient and/or family

1) Describes his or her understanding of extent of disease and current treatment at a level consistent with cultural and educational background and emotional state.

2) Participates in decision making about the plan of care and life activities, if desired or possible.

3) Identifies appropriate community and personal resources that provide information and services.

4) Describes self-care measures and appropriate actions for highly predictable outcomes, oncologic emergencies, and problems associated with the disease, treatment, and side effects of therapy.

5) Describes the treatment schedule when ongoing therapy is predicted.

6) Discusses survivorship issues, advance care planning, and end-of-life care decisions as appropriate.

7) Identifies personal genetic risk factors and implications when indicated.

8) Describes health promotion activities when cancer therapy is complete.

c. Coping

The patient and/or family

1) Communicates feelings about living with cancer.

2) Identifies community resources (e.g., "I Can Cope," Wellness Communities, Cancer Care, Inc., local support groups) that facilitate coping.

3) Uses appropriate personal and community resources and other supportive therapies for managing stress in coping with cancer.

4) Participates in care and ongoing decision making.

5) Communicates feelings about dying.

6) Participates in end-of-life decisions.

7) Identifies alternative resources when present coping strategies do not meet needs.

8) Sets realistic goals that can be accomplished.

9) Contacts the appropriate cancer care team member(s) when faced with difficulties in coping or when social support resources are ineffective.

d. Comfort

The patient and/or family

1) Communicates changes in comfort level using agreed-upon pain/symptom distress rating scale.

2) Describes the source of the discomfort, treatment measures, and expected outcomes.

3) Identifies measures to enhance physical, psychosocial, spiritual, cultural, and environmental factors that increase comfort and promote the continuance of valued activities and relationships.

4) Describes appropriate interventions for potential or predictable problems, such as pain, fatigue, dyspnea, sleep pattern disturbances, nausea, vomiting, and pruritus.

5) Participates in self-care for symptom management.

6) Contacts an appropriate cancer care team member when symptom control is ineffective.

e. Nutrition

The patient and/or family

1) Identifies nutritional measures (e.g., such as a high-fiber, high-protein, and low-fat diet, maintaining ideal weight) that may decrease cancer risk.

2) Identifies measures to prevent or minimize nutritional imbalance.

3) Identifies foods that are appealing and tolerated, as well as those that cause discomfort or are distasteful and unappealing.

4) Describes measures that enhance food intake and retention.

5) Identifies measures to manage anorexia, early satiety, taste changes, mucositis, xerostomia, and nausea and vomiting, if present.

6) Identifies mechanisms to assess his or her nutritional status.

7) Selects appropriate dietary alternatives to provide sufficient nutrients when foods that were part of the customary diet no longer are tolerated.

f. Complementary and alternative therapy

The patient and/or family

1) Reports the use of complementary and alternative therapies.

2) Identifies potential toxicities and food/drug interactions of individual complementary and alternative therapies.

3) Contacts an appropriate cancer care team member if problems associated with complementary and alterative therapies occur.

g. Protective mechanisms

The patient and/or family

1) Identifies factors in personal lifestyle and environment (e.g., smoking cessation, stress reduction, dietary changes, maintaining ideal weight, reducing sun exposure) that may decrease cancer incidence.

2) Lists measures to prevent or minimize infection, bleeding, mucosal trauma, and skin breakdown.

3) Identifies the signs and symptoms of infection, bleeding, mucosal trauma, skin breakdown, and sensorimotor dysfunction.

4) Contacts an appropriate cancer care team member when initial signs and symptoms of infection, bleeding, mucosal trauma, skin breakdown, or sensorimotor dysfunction occur.

5) Describes self-care measures to manage infection, bleeding, mucosal trauma, skin breakdown, and neurologic dysfunction.

h. Mobility

The patient and/or family

1) Explains the impact of fatigue on immobility.

2) Explains the relationship between fatigue and exercise balance.

3) Describes an appropriate management plan to integrate alteration in mobility into his or her lifestyle.

4) Describes optimal levels of activities of daily living in keeping with his or her disease state and treatment.

5) Identifies health services and community resources available for managing changes in mobility.

6) Uses assistive devices to aid or improve mobility.

7) Demonstrates measures to prevent the complications of decreased mobility.

i. Gastrointestinal and urinary function

The patient and/or family

1) Describes appropriate actions when alterations in elimination occur, such as fecal and urinary diversions, fistulas, diarrhea, constipation, bladder insufficiencies, incontinence, dysuria, and fecal or urinary obstruction.

2) Recognizes the importance of adequate elimination for physiological integrity.

3) Identifies and manages factors that may affect elimination, such as diet, stress, physical activity, side effects of treatment, medications, and neurogenic conditions.

4) Develops a plan, within his or her lifestyle, to prevent or manage alterations in elimination.

5) Contacts an appropriate cancer care team member when alterations in elimination occur.

j. Sexuality

The patient and/or family

1) Identifies potential or actual changes in sexuality, sexual functioning, or intimacy (e.g., infertility, dry mucous membranes, alterations in body image, decreased or lack of libido, impotence, early menopause) related to disease and treatment.

2) Expresses feelings about alopecia, body image changes, and altered sexual functioning.

3) Engages in open communication with his or her partner regarding changes in sexual functioning or desire, within cultural framework.

4) Describes appropriate interventions (e.g., sperm banking, consultation with a urologist, sex therapist, or both) for actual or potential changes in sexual function.

5) Identifies other satisfying methods of sexual expression that provide satisfaction to both partners, within cultural framework.

6) Identifies personal and community resources (e.g., "Look Good . . . Feel Better" programs, other support groups) to assist with changes in body image and sexual functioning.

k. Cardiopulmonary function

The patient and/or family

1) Describes plans for daily activity that demonstrate appropriate use of energy to maintain physical activity while minimizing fatigue.

2) Lists measures to reduce or modify pulmonary irritants in the environment, such as smoke, dry air, powders, and aerosols.

3) Describes the effect of environmental extremes on ventilatory function.

4) Describes effective measures to maintain a patent airway.

5) Identifies reasons for altered ventilation, such as disease process, decreased hemoglobin, infection, anxiety, effusion, and an obstructed airway.

6) Identifies an appropriate plan of action if ventilation becomes altered.

7) Identifies signs and symptoms of impaired circulation (e.g., cyanosis, dyspnea, edema).

8) Describes measures to manage altered circulation (e.g., supplemental oxygen, medication).

9) Contacts an appropriate cancer care team member when initial signs and symptoms of change in circulation occur (e.g., fatigue, shortness of breath, dependent edema, other signs of fluid retention).

l. Oncologic emergencies
   The patient and/or family

1) Identifies self-care measures to decrease risk and severity of oncologic emergencies.

2) Identifies signs and symptoms of individualized high-risk emergencies to report to the cancer care team.

3) Identifies strategies to maximize safety.

4) Identifies community resources available for emergency care.

5) Contacts appropriate team member at onset of signs and symptoms of oncologic emergency.

m. Palliative and end-of-life care
   The patient and/or family

1) Participates in end-of-life care and ongoing decision making (as condition permits).

2) Identifies physical, psychosocial, and spiritual concerns that impact suffering.

3) Identifies components of and makes preparations for a "good death."

4) Identifies appropriate pain and symptom management strategies.

5) Identifies meaningful spiritual or religious practices.
6) Identifies specific cultural aspects important to patient or family.
7) Considers hospice as a treatment choice for end-of-life care.

n. Survivorship
The patient and/or family
1) States the potential late effects of cancer treatment and the presenting symptoms.
2) Identifies the potential persistent changes of cancer treatment and related symptom management to optimize quality of life.
3) Participates in long-term follow-up at appropriate intervals.

Standard IV. Planning

The oncology nurse develops an individualized and holistic plan of care that prescribes interventions to attain expected outcomes.

Rationale

A plan of care systematically guides nursing interventions and facilitates the achievement of desired outcomes and continuity of care.

Measurement Criteria

The oncology nurse
1. Bases the plan of care on current knowledge of nursing, evidence-based practice, and biological, sociocultural, behavioral, and physical science.
2. Ensures that the plan of care is patient-centered, outcome-oriented, and based on individualized nursing diagnoses.
3. Incorporates preventive, therapeutic, rehabilitative, and palliative (comforting) nursing actions into the plan of care.

4. Ensures the plan of care reflects sensitivity and respect for the religious, spiritual, social, cultural, and ethnic practices of the patient.
5. Includes individualized physical and psychosocial interventions in the plan of care that are
   a. Supported by current evidence-based research and practice.
   b. Designed to achieve the stated outcomes.
   c. Prioritized according to the patient's needs and preferences.
   d. Culturally competent.
6. Incorporates patient/family education and specific teaching plans related to the 14 high-incidence problem areas into the plan of care.
7. Develops the plan of care in collaboration with the patient, family, and appropriate members of the interdisciplinary cancer care team when possible.
8. Coordinates appropriate resources and consultative services to provide continuity of care and appropriate follow-up in the plan of care.
9. Communicates the plan of care to appropriate members of the interdisciplinary cancer care team.
10. Documents the plan of care in a retrievable form to provide for continuity of care.

Standard V. Implementation

The oncology nurse implements the plan of care to achieve the identified expected outcomes for the patient.

Rationale

The implementation of nursing interventions is designed to promote, maintain, restore, rehabilitate, or palliate the patient's health in congruence with the patient's identified physical, psychosocial, spiritual, and cultural expected outcomes. The overall goal is to influence the patient's overall health, well-being, comfort, and/or quality of life.

Measurement Criteria

The oncology nurse

1. Implements interventions in a timely manner according to the established plan of care.
2. Ensures that interventions are implemented in a safe, culturally competent, appropriate, caring, and humanistic manner.
3. Implements interventions with the concurrence and/or participation of the patient and family when possible.
4. Uses evidence-based research to guide implementation of interventions.
5. Identifies community resources and support systems needed to implement the plan of care.
6. Documents interventions and the patient's responses in the patient's record in a timely manner.

Standard VI. Evaluation

The oncology nurse systematically and regularly evaluates the patient's response to interventions to determine progress toward achievement of expected outcomes.

Rationale

Nursing practice is a dynamic process requiring ongoing evaluation that reflects the patient's health status over time. Evaluation involves the appraisal of nursing diagnoses, interventions, and the plan of care in relation to the patient's health status and expected health outcomes.

Measurement Criteria

The oncology nurse

1. Ensures that the patient/family and the members of the interdisciplinary cancer care team participate collaboratively in the evaluation process when possible.

2. Maintains a systematic and ongoing evaluation process.
3. Collects evaluation data from all pertinent sources.
4. Compares actual findings to expected findings.
5. Reviews and revises the nursing diagnoses, expected outcomes, and plan of care based on the findings of the evaluation process.
6. Uses evidence-based research in the evaluation of expected outcomes.
7. Communicates the patient's response with the interdisciplinary cancer care team and other agencies involved in the healthcare continuum.
8. Documents the findings of the evaluation in the patient's record in a retrievable form, which allows for continuity of care.

Standards of Professional Performance

Standard I. Quality of Care

The oncology nurse systematically evaluates the quality of care and effectiveness of oncology nursing practice within all practice settings.

Rationale

The complex and dynamic nature of the healthcare environment and the evolving findings resulting from evidence-based investigations require oncology nurses to continually appraise how they practice their roles in interdisciplinary care delivery (individually and collectively) and patients' responses to nursing care interventions.

Measurement Criteria

The oncology nurse
1. Participates in quality assessment and improvement activities relative to the nurse's position and practice environment. Such activities may include
   a. Collaborating with other disciplines to determine priority patient care issues for quality when monitoring patient outcomes (e.g., high-incidence problem areas, adverse events, timeliness of treatment, follow-up care, satisfaction with care).
   b. Identifying indicators and outcomes of nurse-sensitive patient care.
   c. Gathering and analyzing data to support the monitoring of oncology nursing care.
   d. Forming recommendations and developing action plans that address options for improving nursing and interdisciplinary care.

    e. Synthesizing the results of evidence-based investigations and integrating findings into practice.

    f. Developing policies and procedures that assimilate the translation of national standards of care into individual practice settings.

2. Solicits feedback from patients and families about their satisfaction with care.

3. Solicits feedback from the interdisciplinary team about nurses' roles in providing care and functioning as a team member.

4. Uses the results of quality monitoring to initiate changes in the practice environment and evaluate the impact of such change.

Standard II. Practice Evaluation

The oncology nurse consistently evaluates his or her own nursing practice in relation to job-specific performance expectations, statewide regulatory requirements, and national oncology nursing professional standards.

Rationale

The oncology nurse is accountable to the lay public and to patients with cancer and, thus, has a responsibility to evaluate his or her practice according to regulations imposed by the work setting, the state of practice, and the professional standards established by the Oncology Nursing Society to ensure safe and competent nursing practice.

Measurement Criteria

The oncology nurse

1. Engages in ongoing performance appraisal with peers, colleagues, and management, identifying strengths, weaknesses, and areas for improvement.

2. Demonstrates and documents competencies relative to specific oncology nurse roles (e.g., an ambulatory chemotherapy nurse can de-clot central venous catheters; an inpatient bone marrow transplant nurse can assess early signs of graft versus host disease within the first 100 days of transplantation; a hospice nurse can recognize and manage dyspnea) and of safety initiatives (e.g., patient identification strategies, early identification of drug-related adverse effects, medication error reduction practice guidelines).
3. Establishes goals for professional development and role maturation.
4. Assists colleagues in evaluating their performance or in seeking assistance with other performance issues (e.g., substance abuse).
5. Serves as a role model or mentor for new oncology nurses.
6. Seeks and encourages oncology nursing certification.

Standard III. Education

The oncology nurse acquires and improves his or her knowledge base related to cancer care and oncology nursing that fosters enhanced competence and critical thinking skills.

Rationale

Learning is a lifelong commitment. Cancer care is characterized by significant and evolving novel innovations in laboratory, behavioral, biological, and technological science that require oncology nurses to remain engaged in continuing educational endeavors.

Measurement Criteria

The oncology nurse
1. Identifies deficits in knowledge and pursues venues (e.g., formal education, clinical experiences, continuing education) to enhance learning.

2. Uses credible, evidence-based oncology educational resources and cites references accordingly.
3. Seeks information outside of oncology sources (e.g., chronic nausea in pregnancy treated with acupressure, fall prevention in patients with dementia, incontinence management strategies with spinal cord–injured patients) and evaluates application to cancer care.
4. Integrates new knowledge and behaviors into practice setting.
5. Develops mentoring, publishing, and presentation skills as appropriate.

Standard IV. Collegiality

The oncology nurse contributes to the professional development of unlicensed and licensed peers and interdisciplinary colleagues.

Rationale

The oncology nurse is responsible for assisting with the provision of new knowledge and skill to all healthcare professionals who provide direct or indirect care to the patient with cancer.

Measurement Criteria

The oncology nurse
1. Creates a practice environment conducive to interdisciplinary excellence.
2. Seeks opportunities for role modeling knowledge and skill in clinical practice.
3. Mentors students and colleagues to expedite specialty knowledge and skill.
4. Participates in the identification of learning needs related to cancer care for members of the interdisciplinary team.
5. Recognizes (formally and informally) contributions of all disciplines in delivering patient care.

6. Participates in collegial peer review focused on the identification of options for future professional development.

Standard V. Ethics

The oncology nurse uses ethical principles as a basis for decision making and patient advocacy.

Rationale

The current environment in which care for patients with cancer is provided is characterized by many ethical dilemmas. These may include withdrawing treatment, withholding treatment, withholding supportive care interventions, advance directives, surrogate decision making, assisted suicide, rationing of care (based on age, cost, and minimal resources), genetic decision making and disclosure, pain management, and use of complementary and alternative therapies.

Measurement Criteria

The oncology nurse
1. Undertakes an inventory of personal beliefs and philosophy regarding quality of life, use of artificial measures to sustain life, what constitutes a "good death," and the use of complementary and alternative therapy approaches.
2. Examines personal spiritual and religious beliefs and degree of cultural competence and their relevance to life and death decision making.
3. Discusses with colleagues ethical dilemmas in cancer care in a nonjudgmental environment of learning and open exchange.
4. Communicates information about advance directives and encourages advance care planning with patients and families.
5. Proactively apprises patients and families of potential ethical issues specific to the individual clinical situation.

6. Maintains patient confidentiality and privacy.
7. Advocates for patients and families in decision-making discussions.
8. Delivers nondiscriminatory care that preserves and protects patient autonomy, dignity, rights, and cultural beliefs.
9. Seeks resources to assist with examination of ethical principles and help formulate ethical decision making.
10. Initiates ethics consultation to assist in solving ethical dilemmas.

Standard VI. Collaboration

The oncology nurse partners with patients, families, the interdisciplinary team, and community resources to provide optimal care.

Rationale

A team is required to provide complex, highly specialized, patient- and family-focused cancer care across the continuum. Through the collaborative process, patients and families are engaged with the cancer care team in sharing their expectations and experiences. The interdisciplinary team uses its specialty knowledge from various disciplines and community resources to assess, plan, implement, and evaluate care.

Measurement Criteria

The oncology nurse
1. Formulates desired outcomes in conjunction with colleagues, patients, and families and evaluates the effectiveness of interventions.
2. Consults with other healthcare providers and makes referrals (e.g., home care, hospice, rehabilitation, palliative care, community-based support groups, and educational offerings) to enhance the patient's cancer experience over time.

3. Participates in the assessment, design, and delivery of educational programs that address multiple healthcare audiences.
4. Offers consultative advice on the improvement of processes in ambulatory, inpatient, homecare, and long-term care services to integrate feedback from multiple providers.
5. Participates in community and political endeavors to improve access to cancer care.

Standard VII. Research

The oncology nurse contributes to the scientific base of nursing practice, education, and management via multiple venues: identifying clinical dilemmas and problems appropriate for rigorous study, collecting data, critiquing existing research, and making use of research.

Rationale

Oncology nurses may be involved in research in various ways depending upon the nurse's role, setting, level of education, and availability of resources (e.g., mentor or researcher consultation, access to literature, allocation of time, availability of grant support, technology to support data analysis).

Measurement Criteria

The oncology nurse
1. Uses evidence-based findings that support the need for changing practice or policy, revising educational approaches, and/or modifying management strategies.
2. Participates in some aspect contributing to the scientific base of cancer nursing practice, including, but not limited to,
   a. Identifying clinical problems suitable for research.
   b. Participating in data collection.

    c. Participating in unit-based, organizational, or community research committees.

    d. Discussing and disseminating the results of research findings with colleagues.

    e. Integrating research findings into the work setting (e.g., policies, procedures, standards and guidelines for patient care).

3. Seeks consultative advice from researchers, statisticians, and other colleagues, as required, to ensure sound research methods and valid study results.

4. Understands rationale for human subject protection in research and requirements for implementing sound research studies.

Standard VIII. Resource Utilization

The oncology nurse considers factors related to safety, effectiveness, and cost in planning and delivering care to patients.

Rationale

Minimization of adverse effects and reduction of error potential are increasingly important to oncology nurses as they advocate for high quality and cost-effective patient care. Care effectiveness may be maximized by delegation and mobilization of the most appropriate resources, which include not only patient and family resources but also community and nationally available resources.

Measurement Criteria

The oncology nurse

1. Evaluates the safety, efficacy, benefits, and burdens associated with intervention options.

2. Undertakes a cost/benefit analysis of proposed interventions with the cancer care team.

3. Triages care requirements based on expertise required to maximize patient outcome.

4. Provides names of community-based resources (e.g., lymphedema and survivor support groups, financial counseling) to assist with continued care requirements.
5. Critiques the quality of existing resources and identifies gaps in resource availability.
6. Advocates for safe staffing levels and ratios.

Standard IX. Leadership

The oncology nurse anticipates the dynamic nature of cancer care and readies herself or himself and colleagues for an evolving future.

Rationale

As the knowledge base, practice environment, and technological resources evolve in cancer care, oncology nurses must respond to, adapt to, and master these changes with an attitude of possibility and innovation rather than one of frustration and resistance.

Measurement Criteria

The oncology nurse
1. Role models critical thinking as it relates to technology transfer and the integration of new practice demands.
2. Assumes responsibility for peer and colleague mentorship in understanding human reactions to change, chaos, and instability in the work environment.
3. Identifies and advocates for vulnerable, underserved populations (e.g., rural elderly patients who do not speak English or use English as a second language, inner-city underserved individuals, single parents with limited or no social support).
4. Anticipates current trends in practice and patient profiles with expectation for continued growth in the future (e.g., ambulatory/home-based care, oncology critical care, technological support

for noninstitutionalized patient assessment and learning via computers and telemonitoring, greater number of long-term cancer survivors, elderly with or at risk for cancer).

5. Integrates an awareness of how decreasing resources impact cancer care in individual work settings.

6. Assists with cost and quality deliberations by translating practice and patient learning requirements associated with new technology.

7. Documents outcomes of oncology nursing intervention and innovation.

8. Demonstrates impact of specialty practice in expert critical thinking, creating novel patient and family education program development, recruiting and retaining oncology nurses, and providing long-term job satisfaction.

Recommended Readings

Aiken, L.H. (1990). Charting the future of hospital nursing. *IMAGE: Journal of Nursing Scholarship, 22*(2), 72–78.

Aiken, L.H., & Patrician, P.A. (2000). Measuring organizational traits of hospitals: The revised nursing work index. *Nursing Research, 49*(3), 146–153.

Bailey, C., Froggatt, K., Field, D., & Krishnasamy, M. (2002). The nursing contribution to qualitative research in palliative care 1990–1999: A critical evaluation. *Journal of Advanced Nursing, 40*(1), 48–60.

Buerhaus, P.I., Needleman, J., Mattke, S., & Stewart, M. (2002). Strengthening hospital nursing. *Health Affairs, 21*(5), 123–131.

Coleman, E.A., Frank-Stromborg, M., Hughes, L.C., Grindel, C.G., Ward, S., Berry, D., et al. (1999). A national survey of certified, recertified, and noncertified oncology nurses: Comparisons and contrasts. *Oncology Nursing Forum, 26*, 839–849.

Dykes, P.C. (2003). Practice guidelines and measurement: State-of-the-science. *Nursing Outlook, 51*(2), 65–69.

Eisenberg, J.M. (1999). Ten lessons for evidence-based technology assessment. *JAMA, 282*, 1865–1869.

Epstein, R.M., & Hundert, E.M. (2002). Defining and assessing professional competence. *JAMA, 287*, 226–235.

Ferrell, B.R., Virani, R., Smith, S., & Juarez, G. (2003). The role of the oncology nurse to ensure quality care for cancer survivors: A report commissioned by the National Cancer Policy Board and Institute of Medicine. *Oncology Nursing Forum, 30*, E1–E11. Retrieved April 6, 2004, from http://www.ons.org/xp6/ONS/Library.xml/ONS_Publications.xml/ONF.xml/ONF2003/FebJan03/Members_Only/Ferrell_article.xml

Giarelli, E., Gholz, R., Haisfield-Wolfe, M.E., Mitchell, A., & Smith, A.M. (2001). SNAP-Shots: Scenes from nursing action plans—The cultivation of leadership in oncology nursing. *Oncology Nursing Forum, 28*, 883–893.

Greene, M.T., & Puetzer, M. (2002). The value of mentoring: A strategic approach to retention and recruitment. *Journal of Nursing Care Quality, 17*(1), 63–70.

Halm, M.A., Gagner, S., Goering, M., Sabo, J., Smith, M., & Zaccagnini, M. (2003). Interdisciplinary rounds: Impact on patients, families and staff. *Clinical Nurse Specialist, 17*(3), 133–142.

Hamric, A.B. (2002). Bridging the gap between ethics and clinical practice. *Nursing Outlook, 50*(5), 176–178.

Holland, J.C. (2001). Improving the human side of cancer care: Psychooncology's contribution. *Cancer Journal, 7*, 458–471.

Howe, H.L., Wingo, P.A., Thun, M.J., Ries, L.A., Rosenberg, H.M., Feigal, E.G., et al. (2001). Annual report to the nation on the status of cancer (1973–1998), featuring cancers with recent increasing trends. *Journal of the National Cancer Institute, 93,* 824–842.

Lee, S.J., Earle, C.C., & Weeks, J.C. (2000). Outcomes research in oncology: History, conceptual framework and trends in the literature. *Journal of the National Cancer Institute, 92,* 195–204.

Mandelblatt, J.S., Ganz, P.A., & Kahn, K. (1999). Proposed agenda for the measurement of quality-of-care outcomes in oncology practice. *Journal of Clinical Oncology, 17,* 2614–2622.

Masys, D.R. (2002). Effects of current and future information technologies on the health care workforce. *Health Affairs, 21*(5), 33–41.

Meyer, G., Foster, N., Christrup, S., & Eisenberg, J. (2001). Setting a research agenda for medical errors and patient safety. *Health Services Research, 36*(1 Pt. 1), x–xx.

Moore-Higgs, G.J., Watkins-Bruner, D., Balmer, L., Johnson-Doneski, J., Komarny, P., Mautner, B., et al. (2003a). The role of licensed nursing personnel in radiation oncology. Part A: Results of a descriptive study. *Oncology Nursing Forum, 30,* 51–58.

Moore-Higgs, G.J., Watkins-Bruner, D., Balmer, L., Johnson-Doneski, J., Komarny, P., Mautner, B., et al. (2003b). The role of licensed nursing personnel in radiation oncology. Part B: Integrating the ambulatory care nursing conceptual framework. *Oncology Nursing Forum, 30,* 59–64.

Morse, J.M., Penrod, J., & Hupcey, J.E. (2000). Qualitative outcome analysis: Evaluating nursing interventions for complex clinical phenomena. *IMAGE: Journal of Nursing Scholarship, 32*(2), 125–130.

Mullan, F. (2002). Time-capsule thinking: The health care workforce, past and future. *Health Affairs, 21*(5), 112–122.

North American Nursing Diagnosis Association. (2001). *Nursing diagnoses: Definitions and classification, 2001–2003.* Philadelphia: Author.

Pasecreta, J.V., & McCorkle, R. (2000). Cancer care: Impact of interventions on caregiver outcomes. *Annual Review of Nursing Research, 18,* 127–148.

Richardson, A., Miller, M., & Potter, H. (2002). Developing, delivering and evaluating cancer nursing services: Searching for a United Kingdom evidence base for practice. *Cancer Nursing, 25,* 404–415.

Smith, C.E. (1999). Caregiving effectiveness in families managing complex technology at home: Replication of a model. *Nursing Research, 48*(3), 120–128.

Smith, T.J., & Hillner, B.E. (2001). Ensuring quality cancer care by the use of clinical practice guidelines and critical pathways. *Journal of Clinical Oncology, 19,* 2886–2897.

Stryer, D., Clancy, C., & Simpson, L. (2002). Minority health disparities: AHRQ efforts to address inequities in care. *Health Promotion Practice, 3*(2), 125–129.

Wilson, R., & Hubert, J. (2002). Resurfacing the care in nursing by telephone: Lessons from ambulatory oncology. *Nursing Outlook, 50*(4), 160–164.

Appendix. Examples of Nursing Diagnoses Used in Oncology Nursing

1. Exchanging
   a. Imbalanced nutrition: less than body requirements, related to nausea and vomiting
   b. Imbalanced nutrition: more than body requirements, related to disease process and treatment
   c. Deficient fluid volume related to disease process and treatment
   d. Risk for infection related to granulocytopenia
   e. Risk for injury related to bleeding
   f. Impaired oral mucous membrane related to radiation therapy/chemotherapy
   g. Impaired skin integrity related to radiation therapy
   h. Constipation related to morphine administration
   i. Impaired urinary elimination: bladder irritation related to chemotherapy
   j. Impaired gas exchange related to lung metastasis
   k. Ineffective breathing pattern related to pleural effusion
   l. Ineffective airway clearance related to laryngectomy
   m. Decreased cardiac output related to previous doxorubicin therapy
   n. Decreased cardiac output related to fluid overload
   o. Risk for injury related to cardiac arrhythmias because of hypokalemia
2. Communicating
   a. Impaired verbal communication related to laryngectomy
3. Relating
   a. Sexual dysfunction related to disease process and treatment
   b. Sexual dysfunction: infertility related to chemotherapy
4. Valuing
   a. Spiritual distress related to cancer diagnosis
5. Choosing
   a. Ineffective coping related to new diagnosis of cancer

    b. Decisional conflict related to cancer treatment options

    c. Compromised family coping related to role changes resulting from disease and treatment

6. Moving

    a. Impaired physical mobility related to lymphedema

    b. Impaired physical mobility related to spinal cord compression

    c. Dressing/grooming self-care deficit related to disease process and treatment

    d. Impaired walking related to peripheral neuropathy

    e. Fatigue related to cancer therapy

    f. Impaired swallowing related to esophagitis from radiation therapy

    g. Disturbed sleep pattern related to chemotherapy administration

7. Perceiving

    a. Disturbed body image related to prostatectomy

    b. Disturbed sensory perception (kinesthetic, tactile) related to peripheral neuropathy

8. Knowing

    a. Deficient knowledge related to prevention and early detection of lung cancer

    b. Deficient knowledge related to prevention and early detection of colon cancer

    c. Deficient knowledge related to prevention and early detection of breast cancer

    d. Deficient knowledge related to disease process

    e. Deficient knowledge related to chemotherapy (or radiation therapy, surgery, biotherapy)

    f. Deficient knowledge related to contraception

    g. Deficient knowledge related to unproven methods of cancer treatment

    h. Impaired memory related to side effects of antiemetic medications used with chemotherapy

9. Feeling

    a. Acute pain related to bone metastasis

b. Pruritus related to carcinoid syndrome
c. Anticipatory grieving related to loss of job after cancer diagnosis and treatment
d. Nausea related to chemotherapy

Note. Based on information from the North American Nursing Diagnosis Association, 2001.